The Caregiver's Guide to

The Cure

The Hero's Journey with Cancer

G. Frank Lawlis, PhD

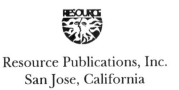

Resource Publications, Inc.
San Jose, California

Editorial director: Kenneth Guentert
Managing editor: Elizabeth J. Asborno
Illustrations: Karen Emenhiser

Reprint Department
Resource Publications, Inc.
160 E. Virginia Street #290
San Jose, CA 95112-5876

Library of Congress Cataloging in Publication Data
Lawlis, G. Frank.
    The caregiver's guide to The cure : the hero's journey with cancer / G. Frank Lawlis.
       p.   cm.
    ISBN 0-89390-274-8
    1. Cancer—Psychological aspects. 2. Storytelling—Therapeutic use. 3. Imagery (Psychology) 4. Stress management. I. Title.
    RC263.L358 1993
    616.99'4'0019—dc20   93-29825

Printed in the United States of America

98 97 96 95 94 | 5 4 3 2 1

Contents

Foreword v

1. How to Use *The Cure* As a Therapeutic Tool . . . 1

2. Symbolic Meanings on the Journey 7

    The Bear

    The Snake

    The Owl

    The Eagle

    The Bull

    The Deer

    The Dolphin

3. Stress, Relaxation, and Conscious Change . . . 19

    Centering Techniques

    Breathing Techniques

Imagery

Meaningfulness of Desire

The Mythic Hero's Journey

4. Self-Empowerment: The Warrior-Self 37

    Life Changes and Skill Demands

    Belief Changes

    Life-Stage Changes

    Life-Rhythm Changes

    Work Changes

    Relationship Changes

    Physical Stamina Changes

Foreword

In *The Cure*, Dr. Lawlis has very skillfully used animal metaphor to communicate important issues of health, illness and life in general that are difficult to express and integrate in other ways. There are several reasons for the problems in relating to these issues, such as fear, identification and attachment.

Some of the most relevant and meaningful in my practice in terms of counseling for health and healing are as follows: the healing influence of the doctor-patient relationship, both positively and negatively; the role of beliefs in health and illness that have underlying spiritual and psychological features; an expanded understanding of the placebo effect in medicine; and the very important role of personal responsibility in physical and psychological health. In an interwoven drama of fear and confusion between Alex and his relationships, the ultimate existential struggle for meaningfulness evolves in similar processes I have observed in my patients.

The helpful skills required for the successful interaction with one's disease is very effectively communicated in *The Cure*, with its intricacies of complex feelings of ignorance, pride and possessiveness. The defined skills used in my practice that are specific to *The Cure* are: the role of relaxation, and centering oneself in health; the health value of self nurturing; the physical, mental and spiritual aspects of disease; the important role of the family and support in health. Dr. Lawlis has used animal characters, freeing the reader to learn the important lessons with little likelihood of personal identification and attachment that could interfere with objectivity.

The problem of medical politics and the many difficulties in using the current medical system in present day is shown in many ways, like the mythical hero's journey where the current health care system is like a dark and unknown forest of past mythic stories. All come together to make this a clear, charming, informative and healing book.

O. Carl Simonton, MD, author of
Getting Well Again *and* The Healing Journey

1. How to Use *The Cure* As a Therapeutic Tool

The value of a good story is its ability to provide a path, perhaps a mythical one, through one of life's obstacles. Sometimes stories reveal sources of hope, others relate specific skills, and others may teach cultural knowledge. Examples come from virtually all of the spiritual traditions of the world, some of which are best known through biblical tradition, such as the Prodigal Son or Job. Fairy tales are re-told not only because they are entertaining but because they are remembered for the subtle wisdom they impart. In "Cinderella," perhaps the wisdom communicated is the knowledge of spiritual supervision or the ultimate good of pure motivation. In "Jack and the Beanstalk," the wisdom could be in the positive messages of cleverness and courage in the face of authoritarian unfairness.

Whatever moral or implicit messages are relevant to the listener, the impact of a story can last a lifetime.

The Cure: The Hero's Journey with Cancer is a story about a specific path in healthcare that most of us may have to learn at some time in our lives. I have found its significance to be relevant to adults and children alike as they confront the enormous tasks of dealing with the medical care of catastrophic diseases, such as cancer, cardiovascular trauma, chronic pain, paralysis, and others. Perhaps the health system is relatively new in human existence; hence very few stories relate to the mystery and confusion of being thrown into the medical culture. Health care people use a different language and wear different clothes; being in the role of patient is different from any other. Just as the forest in many stories represents a dark and fearful place, the hospital in contemporary times represents a frightening situation.

It is important to remember that this story is not about modern medicine and its treatment. There are sensitive and insensitive doctors, nurses, and other healthcare people. Although Alex deals with many of the less sensitive ones as part of his path, it is important to remember that Alex's ultimate decision was to return to the medical system and learn from the respective wisdoms of all the healthcare professionals, once he could realize the human limitations of perceptions. The metaphoric characters represent different considerations on the personal health path, and, as we will see in the upcoming sections, they will relate to the personal imprints of each of our histories and reactions to realities.

The medical healthcare system is a human-made mystery based upon the development of technologies and professional specialty training as well as the economies of healthcare costs and management. Consequently, the

2

involvement of a layperson typically includes confusion and frustration. Moreover, because of the post-World War II romantic attachment to the technology of medicine, the power of the media has often further separated the cloistered sanctuary of hospital care into a sacred, "not to be questioned" atmosphere. There the priestesses and priests of cure work with sterile and objective intentions, without a great deal of input from the ignorant citizenry.

Critical disease is a major source of stress to anyone, and the threat of death or debilitating conditions can be enough to enhance major coping mechanisms to the maximum. However, the combination of entering into the maze of a confusing healthcare system and the personal turmoil of dealing with a disease often defeat the spirit of the patient and the family before a treatment can begin. The person's new role as "the victim" of a biological trauma crosses over into social settings as well.

The wolf-dog symbol in this story is not used by accident as our guide on the journey toward health. One of the symbolizations of the wolf-dog icons by many of the primitive cultures of the world has been one as a guide and teacher. The use of these animals as seeing-eye companions and in police support also confirms their potential aid to humankind in this regard. The Zuni tradition labels the following characteristics of the wolf:

- Loyalty
- Insight and Revelation
- Social Values
- Teaching and Learning

- Clarity

- Inner Guidance

- Expression

- Newness, New Choices

The falcon is often recognized as a symbol of a messenger of oracles, given to providing omens. The Zuni tradition characterizes the raven with these powers:

- Magic

- Transformational Powers

- Courage and Comfort

- Guidance into Shadow Side

The relationship between the wolf and raven is a loving relationship in which a dialogue can be expressed. The other animal figures have like symbolic values that have relevance to human values and concerns; these will be discussed on the journey.

Using story for therapeutic purposes benefits listeners through the multi-levels of communication. At the basic level of communication, there is the metaphoric journey through personal obstacles toward the meaningfulness of disease. At this level, the storyteller merely tells the story, allowing the listener to relate the elements of the tale to his or her personal life, at either a conscious or unconscious level of appreciation.

On the second and third levels, the teller relates the story with a more interpersonal relationship between him or herself and the listener. At these levels, the teller takes on more responsibility in serving as a facilitator and guide for the listener's process.

Relating the story on the second level of communication, the teller takes on the role of an educator. He or she can impart the information about the story symbols, learned either from this guide or from personal experience, especially as they relate to current situations that arise in the healing process. Such teaching can be accomplished both verbally and non-verbally.

In telling the story, the teller will have many opportunities to teach the listener how to deal with the stress of disease or medical interventions; options for using breathing techniques or imagery are discussed in chapter 3. Perhaps using either or both the written relaxation and imagery scripts of the book or accompanying instruction tape, the storyteller can train the listener in the skills of relaxation and breathing techniques, especially in preparation for stress-inducing events such as painful drug administrations or nausea-producing situations.

Perhaps the most difficult yet most powerful way to tell the story is to use the non-verbal modeling effect. The storyteller models the relaxation and breathing techniques by the way he or she *tells* the story, thereby communicating the use of the techniques without actually going through the steps. Because the storyteller is often a family member or a close friend, it is difficult to remain relaxed and calm in the face of impending discomfort for the patient. However, patients often respond to novel events by reacting to the behavior of those close around them. Therefore, the storyteller needs to be aware that he or she can affect the response of the listener in either a positive or negative way. I strongly recommended that the storyteller spend some time with him or herself to develop a relaxing and calm tone in the voice, demonstrating deep breathing patterns while telling the story. The storyteller should be willing to retell the relaxation portion of the story several times, implicating the relaxation response and skill to stressful times or in preparation for imagery process.

Inherent in the educational process is the dolphin's imagery explanation about the physical characteristics of the immunity forces within the body. Although imagery will be discussed later in this book, the awareness of inner protective forces does have positive impact upon a person's response to medical treatment, and the information does not detract from other medical discussions or descriptions. In fact, it may be helpful to describe the specific medical treatment at the cellular level so that the patient can understand the expected outcomes of the treatments; then he or she can participate in the imagery process.

The third level of communication involves the teller acting in the role of the falcon, traveling with the listener through his or her experience on the journey. The listener can tell new stories or share different responses to the animals. Different experiences in the healthcare system can be related or even negated through a discussion about each. In a sense, the storyteller can learn a new story. Most important is that the teller be a friend and comrade as the listener evolves on the personal path.

Levels of Interaction
between Storyteller and Listener

Level One	Storyteller gives story content without personal involvement
Level Two	Storyteller serves as educator, verbally and non-verbally
Level Three	Storyteller serves as friend/ listener, creating a personal myth, new story

2. Symbolic Meanings
on the Journey

As Joseph Campbell once remarked, "Myths are clues to the spiritual potentialities of the human life." Stories are told to try to come to terms with the world and to harmonize our lives with our realities. The story of Alex's *search* for the meaning of his disease (and eventual decision to *live* the experience of that meaning) includes some basic symbolic features that may be meaningful at a genetic or archetypal level. These symbols may be cultural or personal, but in my experience they have been used for healing in many primitive communities and have evoked responses from patients I have worked with over the years. Nevertheless, many of the symbols have multiple meanings, and I acknowledge that my usage is not universal. Therefore, I recommend changing the symbolic host to a more meaningful one if doing so will maintain the basic story theme for the teller's particular listener.

The following interpretations of the symbolic characters are basic to the story of Alex; the underlying dynamics are crucial to anyone's path toward health. These are presented as aids to the storyteller as an educator to the listener (the second level of communication explained in chapter 1).

The Bear

Probably one of the most frequent totems in Native American lore, the bear often represents strength and stamina. Its hibernatory habits introduce the wisdom in the realms of sleep and dreaming. The bear also represents an ultimate authority with which Alex is dealing in terms of his future. The major message from the bear is that he has a diagnosis, and nothing is to be discussed in terms of its validity or reliability.

In the mythical interaction with authority, each person has to become the authority of his or her own destiny, and from the first chapter on, Alex gives his authority away. This response is common and understandable. When there is pain and probable loss of function or appetite, we search for an authority to explain the problem with the hope of "fixing it." We are glad to give our cars, television sets, our bank accounts, and even our bodies to those experts who have clarity about the prob-

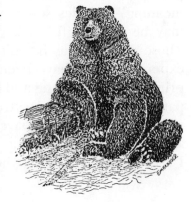

lems and promise to remedy the situation as soon as possible.

We begin our journey by searching for an authority who will explain our problem in a relevant metaphor, and who will cure the part inside us that is hurting us. Although it is wise to seek out those with great resources, it is important to remain responsible and clear about our own destiny.

After telling the story, the teller could possibly extend it by having Alex return to the bear with the intention of participating as an equal in the healthcare team. He could exercise his choice of using the bear's wisdom without giving the final choice to the bear. Hopefully, listeners will learn to deal with authority in a positive way, rather than either denying the wisdom or fearing the responsibility of dealing with power.

The Snake

Since the earliest times in recorded history, the snake has been seen as a healer that comes from the deepest part of the world with its wisdom. The early Greeks and many Native Americans and Mayans used snakes in direct interventions, apparently with great success. In biblical stories, the snake was the giver of special wisdom and a tool used by Moses. However, the snake's power can be used in many ways, and in Alex's and the snake's initial confrontation, Alex is confronted with his own inherent

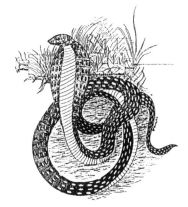

destructive forces. By using the metaphor of "ants eating the inside" for the disease, the snake relates to the ongoing forces within that are gnawing away. These forces can be feelings or worries that constantly bother us but which we push into the back of our mind. Yet these forces cannot be dismissed. An example is the Boss who says something that hurts our feelings in a significant way, but we choose not to deal with the Boss. Yet the feeling constantly eats away at our consciousness the rest of the day or week or until we decide to express our feelings.

For example, I met a man who carried the guilt of an untimely comment for years. He had complimented his sister about the shape of her legs one day, but she took it the wrong way and accused him of trying to destroy her self-esteem. They had not talked about it for years, but he had always thought that the social distance between them was the result of that one comment and had never forgiven himself. When he finally discussed it with her, he discovered that she had forgotten the incident and had been relating the social distance to his shyness.

All too often our problems are blamed upon our own internal forces, and although the person pointing out this blame may be correct and perceptive (as the snake), he or she may suggest that our only path is to kill that part of ourselves, with surrounding parts getting killed as well. The solution becomes a partial suicide, with the hopes that the best part of us survives. With regard to cancer cells, we must find a way of destroying the enemy, but we must also recognize our own power and goodness.

In the storytelling, the teller should emphasize that, in the interaction between Alex and the snake, the snake does not help Alex perceive his own goodness. Again, our source of wisdom and support is our awareness that the self is in a positive process. We must identify who the real enemy is and rally the positive forces. If there are evil ants, there must be good ants who can fight for the self.

The Owl

The owl enjoys a broad reputation among the early cultures of America and Europe. Some interpret the presence of the owl as an omen of death and something to be feared. Others interpret the owl as a sign of changing luck and good fortune. Probably because of its nighttime hunting habits, this creature maintains an aura of dark mystery. However, the owl consistently seems to symbolize a time of upcoming transition. Certainly it is true that Alex will be going through a major transition, one way or another.

This part of Alex's journey introduces sin as a source of disease. The original definition of sin is derived from an archery term: the distance by which the arrow misses the target. In the most generic sense, the greater our distance from the path we are supposed to travel, the greater our sin.

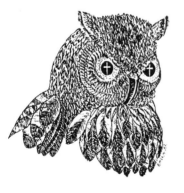

The problem is in defining the personal path for any one individual, and according to all religions that speak to this process, only the relationship of the person to their spiritual consciousness can determine what that path might be. Many paths exist for dif-

11

ferent individuals, and if one of the reasons for the direction in our journey is to teach us spiritual lessons, who are we to question the mind of God?

In many ways Alex's disease ultimately provides some method of learning his spiritual path; however, Alex must first learn to deal with being diagnosed as sinful and then develop a boundary against assault from another person. The diagnosis of having a disease, any disease, makes us especially vulnerable to any individual who proclaims healthiness as an outgrowth of his or her relationship with God. A sort of shame is inherit in being sick or diagnosed with a disease. Perhaps this response recalls the days of being "unclean, hence unholy." Another way that I understand the association between sin and disease is the meaningfulness of pain as punishment. From our childhood days of learning right from wrong with physical punishment as a motivator, we associate the feeling of pain with being punished. Hence, we begin to wonder what wrongdoing has occurred to cause the resulting pain. This kind of associated thinking is very common in most of the patients I have worked with over the years.

The storyteller should be alert to this association and be ready to offer some support in separating the disease from moral criticisms. The owl offers Alex a superficial meaningfulness to his spiritual path, and although Alex ultimately rejects the moral judgment, he also begins to understand that disease is an opportunity to learn about his spiritual journey at some level of understanding. Therefore, in a strict sense, disease can help guide us along our spiritual path and reduce the "sin" or distance from that path; however, the listener should be aware that the journey is always a personal one and cannot be judged by anyone else. A true spiritual helper is there to help us along our path—not criticize our unfortunate position.

The Eagle

In both American and European literature, the eagle is consistently considered a totem of great significance. In Celtic tradition eagles have qualities of swiftness, keen sight and magic. For example, there is the Eagle of Cilgwry, whose power leads to the finding of the Celtic god Mabon. In the Irish text *The Voyage of Maelduin*, an ancient eagle renews itself in a lake, an act representative of the renewal of wisdom in every generation. In many Native American traditions, the eagle is the link between the Heavens and Earth, similar to the Thunderbird, and carries messages to and from humans and gods.

In Alex's story, the eagle represents the psychological aspects of our self, the pathos of the psyche. The wolf is confronted with a Freudian or psychosomatic metaphor of disease, which explains how the development of disease might be the substitution for a primal need of the mind. Research has demonstrated that stress does, in fact, diminish immunity and may create the opportunity for disease; however, the eagle gives his own interpretation of Alex's dynamics instead of helping Alex develop his own understanding. The obstacle Alex has to overcome again is the externalization of what he is and the unique personality that he is. Too often a little scientific support promotes

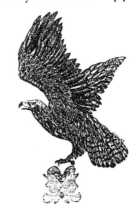

a whole sea of pat and stereotypical explanations that tend to be overgeneralized to apply to all people, and the wisdom of the individual relationships is lost.

The storyteller must clarify, if questioned, that the listener is to look within him or herself to understand the connections between the body and the mind in terms that can be understood for the self. There is very important information about the links between body and mind, which could be useful to know for healthcare; the dolphin explains those relationships later. In this chapter, the eagle does not provide that information in a meaningful way.

The Bull

The bull or ox does not appear broadly in literature about possible interpretations of its presence. Generally speaking, the bull or ox represents brute strength and determination in accomplishment of specific goals. It is seen as an ally in performing difficult tasks, similar to the Blue in the Paul Bunyan stories and myths.

Consistent with that interpretation, the bull confronts Alex with a determined program of physical exercise to

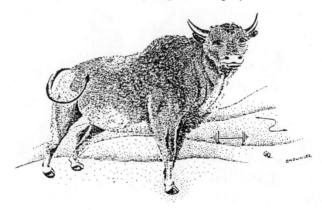

help him with his disease. What the bull discusses has its special validity in the sense that physical exercise is helpful, both physically and mentally, in the management of disease. Moderate exercise helps immunity factors, increases healing potentials and decreases depression. Alex admits that he does feel better; however, like all treatments, the fitness regimen is not the minor alteration in life habits that will have the greatest effect on health. An overall change that includes the body and the mind and the spirit makes the difference. Alex comes to this conclusion at the end of the story, but at this time he is confronted with this piecemeal explanation.

Bulls are not known for their wisdom or intelligence, so, if necessary, the teller may advise the listener about how narrow-minded some people can be about their ideas of healthcare. This applies not only to healthcare professions but also to allied health non-professionals and ex-patients. For example, the patient who believes that he or she was cured by Treatment X (regardless of the name), may be over-enthusiastic about its application to everyone else.

The Deer

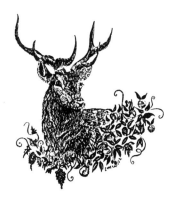

In mythology literature, probably no totem has more words written to describe it than the deer. The deer was always seen as a magical creature that could lead one into the Otherworld. In Celtic myths, the deer often appears in the guise of a beautiful woman who can re-take the shape of the deer at will. Many Native American tribes, such as the Huichole, see the deer as a central part of the whole community's spiritual practices—a kind of "deer cult." Knowing these legends, it is easy to understand why the myth of Santa Claus integrates the use of reindeer to soar into the heavens for magical travel feats.

Alex meets the deer after much frustration on his travels, and he once again has to deal with a source of wisdom which is not incorrect but has too narrow an implication for the individual. Nutrition is very important in healthcare, especially in the treatment and prevention of some cancers; however, nutrition is specific to a person. Men and women require different diets. People living in different climates require different diets. People living under different stress levels, working under different conditions, and even sleeping in different time zones require different diets. Therefore, to specify one and only one nutritional regimen for the entire animal kingdom is too restricted.

The teller can recommended that the listener listen to his or her own body and become aware of what feels correct based on his or her energy level. The listener may also learn about what goes into the body for energy use. It may be important to change the diet as part of the total life change.

The Dolphin

Hawaiian Shamans speak of the dolphin much like other traditions speak of the eagle: possessing great wisdom that comes from deities. However, instead of from messengers from above, the dolphins have sources

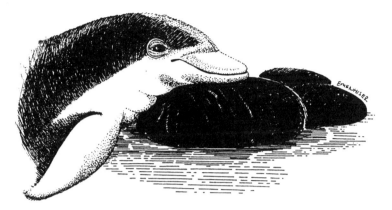

from the underworld or undersea, similar to the eel or snake.

In this regard Alex has the opportunity to receive information about the connections of the mind and body and spirit in a loving way. Perhaps the symbolism is too obvious that this first feminine figure is also the first to demonstrate consideration for Alex as an individual. However, the story is not to indict male healthcare professionals or the various healthcare practices. The discrimination in the approaches, similar to the discrimination in L. LeShan's *The Mechanic and The Gardener*, is to highlight the nature of caregiving and to humanize the path in healthcare.

If the patient can learn to be sensitive to him or herself, recognizing the possible obstacles in the healthcare system as opportunities for growth, then the experience can be a positive one. After all, the mythic journey is for the growth of the person with the disease, not necessarily for the growth of the healthcare system. The system is what it is, and it may undergo changes one way or another, but it will ultimately be the responsibility of the individual to learn the lessons, whatever conditions exists.

3. Stress, Relaxation, and Conscious Change

From a physical and mental perspective, there are few sources more destructive to the body than ongoing stress. Stress can be defined in a multitude of ways. For example, one definition of stress is "the action on a body of any system of balanced forces whereby strain results."[1] In physiology, stress can be defined as "any stimulus that disturbs or interferes with the normal physiological equilibrium of an organism."[2] Both definitions share a central focus, that stress is an imbalance or disharmony in the forces within and external to the body or person.

The manifestations of stress come mainly in three forms: physiological, cognitive and behavioral. The

---

1 *American Heritage Dictionary* (New York: Dell, 1983).
2 Mark Schwartz, *Biofeedback* (New York: Guilford Press, 1987), 64.

physiological aspects are those functions of the body that respond to alarms or crisis states of fear. The eye pupils dilate, the heart beats faster, the blood pressure rises, muscles become tense, adrenal hormones begin surging, etc. Although these functions do have some adaptive reactions to those situations in which we need immediate responses, such as dealing with an oncoming train or dealing with a storm, continuous stimulation will eventually and quickly exhaust the entire bodily system. When the crisis state is not appropriate or the system becomes exhausted, the body becomes vulnerable to other problems. For example, the immunity system also becomes fatigued, pain insulating neuropeptides become less efficient, and the body becomes generally weaker.

The cognitive aspects relate to the interpretation of reality by the individual. As stress mounts with little or no release, people often begin to lose their self-confidence in dealing with life problems. This tendency may relate to fatigue or decreased capacities to think and problem-solve efficiently. One of the theories is that the fear or anxiety response is to minimize breathing patterns, similar to an animal paralyzed by fear, waiting in brush for the danger to pass. In our modern culture, however, people can't tell when their stressful situations will pass. Without a clear timeframe for holding our breath, tensing our muscles, etc., we eventually deplete the oxygen supply in our brains. Consequently, we have less energy and resources for dealing with problems; with less capacity, the problems tend to multiply—at least, they seem to grow larger.

The behavioral component is probably an outgrowth of the processes begun in the first two. As we have weaker bodies and less mental flexibility, we tend to act inappropriately. It is well known that people with high levels of stress tend to have more accidents, make more mistakes in business and behave more destructively in interpersonal relationships such as marriages.

Stress has been determined to contribute to the onset of a variety of diseases—namely, heart disease, cancer, arthritis and strokes; however, stress *resulting from* being diagnosed with such diseases is extremely common, and managing that stress level important to the management of the disease. When one is under high stress conditions, the success of medical interventions is compromised; medications can become difficult to administer appropriately because of unpredictable reactions. Consequently, it is useful to learn skills to deal with stress. In the following section, specific tools are described as approaches for stress management; these are also described in the story, and practical approaches are offered on the accompanying tapes. If appropriate, the storyteller might engage in direct skill development.

Centering Techniques

Before the storyteller begins a story, especially one with a theme of comfort and support such as *The Cure*, he or she should find a center within the self from which to express him or herself. If the expression comes from a place of fear or insecurity, the underlying message will be fear and insecurity. Accomplishing this may be difficult in times of crisis or fear about the person's condition. The teller's primary concern is to prepare the person to listen, to comfort him or her in the midst of turmoil, and to create a place of sacred space, even in our busy world.

There are many centering approaches, and the teller does not have to dedicate a great deal of time to this process. The important step is to develop a sensitivity toward the self, relaxing any tension that may compromise the impact of the story. One centering exercise that may be helpful is to develop a brief meditative or prayerful script that the teller could verbalize or process quietly as a prelude to the story, such as the following:

> Instead of thinking about telling a story in this place, let's close our eyes and think about another place. Let's think about telling a story in a very quiet place, a place where everything is very calm, and we can really listen to the story. The place would be very quiet and restful, maybe in a meadow, or in your bed, or in a favorite place that you could tell me about. Let us take a moment or two and just think about being in a very peaceful place, so that we can get very relaxed and can listen to everything about the story.

Breathing Techniques

In the management of anxiety, pain and nausea, simple breathing techniques have proven to be profoundly useful. One of the most popular and effective has been the "puff" or "blow" technique. The idea is to exhale puffs of air in rapid succession when discomfort or nausea comes into consciousness. Oftentimes, a patient is told to "blow the pain away" with the breath. This technique is always accompanied by the instructions to relax while the blowing or puffing is going on, so that a sense of mastery over the pain or nausea is accomplished; additionally, a sense of mastery over the anxiety of non-control is associated with this approach. This is not unlike the birthing techniques described in literature on natural birthing.

Another breathing technique directly described in the story is the rhythmic breathing cycle or "circle breathing." The simplest way to instruct this approach is to demonstrate breathing in and out in even intervals of time, usually counting specific numerals or reciting specific phrases with each inhalation or exhalation. For example, I usually count to seven with each phase of breathing to determine an even interval of time elapsing in each cycle. So, the process would be to breathe in, counting "1...2...3...4...5...6...7," then release the breath, counting "1...2...3...4...5...6...7," and so forth. The patient may feel dizzy in the beginning, but this feeling will subside and the resultant relaxation response should begin to emerge into consciousness.

Often the person is more comfortable reciting a phrase with each inhalation and exhalation, such as, "In every day I am getting better and better," or something more personal. As long as the person is using the same phrase for both the in and out breaths, it should work.

Although the process can become boring and other events can easily detract from the progression, I highly recommended continuing the breathing for at least ten minutes for effect. Following are other suggestions for phrases to say on the in and out breaths, which can help in relaxation and pain reduction:

On the Inhalation	On the Exhalation
I close my eyes	and bring my awareness inside.
I deepen my breathing	and quiet my thoughts.
I allow my body to be still	and relax my muscles.
I open my heart	and free my spirit.
I flow with life;	I am one with all.

In terms of modifying a stress reaction, breathing is our most accessible physical behavior for the management of stress. Consequently, it is the most appropriate for the general case of anxiety management. Remember that this cycle of breathing is the attempt to reach some harmony, bringing it back into the system. Therefore, calm and soothing tones of support are critical to the technique.

Imagery

As a person begins to focus attention upon any part of the body, physiological change usually takes place. Often blood circulation changes; sometimes other biochemical changes occur, such as an increase of neuropeptides and endorphins, which begin to insulate the body against pain and alert the immune system to guard against invasion. Nevertheless, the idea relevant to telling this story is that the mental pictures we form about our bodies and minds can help us cope more effectively with the disease and the anxiety surrounding it. We may approach this with an eye toward both educating ourselves about the disease and taking action in the process.

By becoming educated about the disease, we can gain a more realistic picture of what's happening, rather than let our imagination go. Not only will we get a better understanding of the problem, we can get an idea of how to defeat it. For example, as someone with folliculitis feels the discomfort in his or her head and hears the diagnosis, he or she may conjure a multitude of images out of fear and lack of knowledge about the language of medicine. However, once educated about the disease, he or she becomes aware that "folliculitis" simply refers to inflammation and possible infection of the hair follicles. Since this condition is probably not terminal or even chronic, the person's initial fear of major life change or disfigurement will likely lessen.

The next step is to participate in the healing process. In the case of the person with folliculitis, managing—and curing—that disease requires educating that person about consistently cleaning the skin and developing stress management skills. Thus, after getting a clear image of how the disease may be cured, the person takes a responsible position of action in the healing process and can eventually take credit for his or her eventual recovery.

One of the important lessons Alex learns is that his personal symbols can empower him in his disease management and will perhaps help him transcend much of his frustration in the process. To most people, disease seems to be a dis-empowering process, often interrupting life plans and visions. As we develop our image of the disease, perhaps we will recognize a relationship between previous events in our life and the disease. For example, focusing our energy upon buying a new house *might* have been a factor in the development of physiological symptoms, or a divorce *might* have caused those headaches. Understanding how disease might relate to our life circumstances adds to our sense of control.

As the patient learns more about the physical and psychological aspects of a disease, the caregiver could recommend that the person investigate what healing symbols are important to him or her and integrate these symbols into an ongoing healing imagery. From time to time, I have patients draw what healing symbols emerge for them. Some draw the sun; others draw power animals, such as the deer or dolphin. Whatever is drawn or described can be included as part of the relaxation or breathing exercises, especially when experiencing medical interventions. For example, it is appropriate to imagine the healing and relaxing powers of the sun as one is undergoing radiation or spinal taps.

I have also found it meaningful to educate patients through a visual exercise of drawing the components (the cells, the medicine, etc.) in order to recruit the patients' efforts in their own treatment. As indicated in the story, Alex could participate on his path toward health only after he understood the underlying forces of the disease and could relate them to his own life. This principle has been demonstrated over and over again in research journals: patients who have a clear understanding of their disease and the strategies underlying the medical treatment do better and with less anxiety than those patients who are confused.

One example relevant to the process of a person teaching his or her body new ways of reacting or changing comes from the field of sports psychology. We know that in order for a person to learn a new sport or activity, such as riding a bicycle or playing tennis, two stages have to occur in the process. In the first stage, the person forms a clear image of the event. They may have observe the act by watching others, or they may have heard about the process enough so that a clear image appears. For example, by watching other people play basketball, a person's mind begins to program the body according to the image portrayed. Interestingly, the research findings indicate that poor models create poor habits; watching a poor driver tends to produce poor driving students, so there is some wisdom in selecting the proper models to create images.

The second stage in the process is to provide for a period of time for trial and error. If a person is learning to throw basketballs through a hoop, he or she will miss the hoop many times, but if the person can maintain the image of success and not become self-critical, he or she will eventually be able to develop the skill of basketball throwing. In this training, it is important for both caregiver and patient to not become stressed and impatient. Given the possible negative effects of stress on performance, a person's image of success can become confused and evolve into an image of defeat or failure.

This self-defeating attitude occurs all too often, especially in the United States. We expect too much of ourselves too quickly. As we experience mistakes, we want to dismiss ourselves as "stupid" or "clumsy," with such admissions supposedly covering up our embarrassment. We become our worst critic, comparing ourselves to others in appropriate ways. When the great golfer Arnold Palmer was asked to comment on how he could make so much money by merely swinging a golf club a few times on a weekend, he replied that no one paid him for the million times he practiced each swing of each golf club before he achieved the sufficient skill to compete professionally. It takes a Buddhist monk two years isolated in a cave just to learn the art of breathing. Practice is important to learning any skill; if the person is patient, the skill will come.

Our engagement with disease involves this trial-and-error process at times. We do not know what specific image, life change, or even medical interventions will cause an improvement in health. That is the message in the story of Alex: life is a mystery and there are many paths to follow. Some of these paths may be constructive and productive; some may not be relevant to an individual during a particular phase of life. The important thing is to continue the mission, searching without blaming the self or others and maintaining the appropriate image or goal within one's mind.

There are many imagery approaches. Some relate to the visual sense, seeing things when the eyes are closed. Some relate to the auditory sense, hearing songs or words in the mind. All the senses can be incorporated into a total imagery process. One of the best examples for relaxation imagery is the "Tub Experience." The script is as follows:

> Take a moment and begin to relax with your eyes closed. Allow your breathing to relax you more and more. As you continue to breathe... deeply...and rhythmically, feel the air filling every cell in your body, making you feel lighter and lighter.
>
> Now imagine yourself relaxing comfortably... in a bubbling hot springs...or in a hot tub or whirlpool....The steaming water enfolds and surrounds you...all the way to your chin.... Everything is safe and you are very secure.... The water is gently massaging your skin...with millions of tiny bubbles...that caress you, and cleanse you...draining away your tension...and troubles....You can feel free.
>
> Enjoy the warmth...and comfort...and support...of the water. *(Pause.)*
>
> Notice how your skin tingles...how your face feels full...how the pores all over your body open up to the healing warmth of the bubbling water. *(Pause.)*
>
> Listen to the sound of the bubbles...as they percolate through the water...and gurgle to the surface....Every part of your body is totally relaxed...supported by the warm water and tiny bubbles....Your arms and legs...may feel heavy...and warm...and relaxed...yet floating to the top of the water. The warmth of the water

penetrates every part of the body...allowing you to unwind...and let go....Allow the cleansing warmth of the water...to drain away any tension or discomfort that you are feeling....Watch the tension evaporate...as the bubbles rise to the surface...leaving you totally in peace....Stay and enjoy the warmth and relaxation of the water....Enjoy the feelings of comfort...and calm...for as long as you wish. (Pause.)

When you are ready...return to your routine of the day...refreshed...revitalized...unworried... taking the peace of this place...with you.

The accompanying cassette tape gives instructions about the potential use of imagery in conjunction with the story, especially in chapter seven. After listeners have a grasp of the dynamics of the disease, I often ask them to make up a similar story, including their personal symbols of healing, the education about their treatment, and their personal path.

Meaningfulness of Desire

As depicted in the story of Alex, disease can be a teacher. The physical dynamics of disease can be a story unto themselves, sometimes fitting into the social and psychological spheres of the person's life. When the disease is serious or life threatening, it is not unusual for the listener to begin to ask the basic questions: "Why am I here? What is my mission in life? What is my life supposed to mean?" These questions often frighten family members and friends because they are confused as to why they are emerging. Actually, this is a particularly important time to consider these questions because if the disease affects part of a lifestyle or process (such as work habits, eating habits, etc.), then something is going to die or be transformed so that the person can become healthy and in harmony again. Something will change if the disease is going to change, and it is time to begin some value clarification.

For example, consider the man who has just survived a heart attack. He has been a hard-working man who has smoked two packs of cigarettes a day for all of his adult life. He has typically eaten meals of fifty percent fat content and has never learned to relax for five minutes at any one time. The heart attack is probably part of his lifestyle, and to begin a life more in harmony with health, something will have to die—either some of his habits or his whole body. Now, the smoking, eating, working too hard, etc., may be problematic to change because these habits did not exist just because they were begun. These habits and all lifestyle behaviors have value. Working hard certainly has great value to self-esteem. Smoking may relate to another aspect of self-esteem, occasionally described as personal control issues. It is very difficult to change a lifestyle, even in the face of major threat, without a reason for doing so. Internal dialogue about what purpose our lifestyles serve is termed in this book as "the spiritual basis of life." Unless this man (or Alex) comes to terms with the deeper issues of what life means to be lived, and if he continues to pursue his values in the old way, the disease will continue to erode the physical fibers of strength and will ultimately complete the cycle. That is what is meant by "learning through the disease." What does it have to teach us? What new values are we to consider? What avenues of obtaining these values are available?

One of the methods for finding personal answers to life is to go on a vision quest, a journey to a special place where we can open the heart and mind to become receptive to any psychological or spiritual information. However, it is also possible to go on an imagery vision quest, thereby making it feasible to obtain important answers to some of these existential issues in a more timely manner. The accompanying vision quest cassette tape provides a general approach to the steps of a vision journey; however, the tape may be too structured with time limits and specific imagery for some individuals. Therefore, it might be more helpful for the caregiver to instruct the person about the general phases of the journey and allow the person to conduct his or her own vision quest, applying his or her symbols or metaphors to the imagery experience. The phases of the journey are as follows:

1. **Formulating the mission or question:** In order to make the best use of this journey, before beginning the venture the person should determine a question or reason for the trip. The more specific and relevant the question is, the more relevant and specific the answer will be. The thought must be formulated before the journey begins and held throughout the travel.

2. **Departing from this reality:** If there is a need for a journey, it is to travel to another place; therefore, some form of departure is required. The tape gives the choice of traveling through the earth (as in a tunnel or cave), through the sky (as in flying by oneself or on a bird, or by being lifted on smoke or a cloud), or through water (on a boat or by the current of a river). Other possible forms of departure include climbing a tall tree to the heavens or riding a magical animal or carpet.

3. **Finding a sacred place:** Sooner or later, the ultimate conclusion of a journey is to find a place to stop. This place should be peaceful and welcoming, like a meadow or a home. It is the responsibility of the person to determine this place by the description of its atmosphere and feeling rather than by its actual prescribed characteristics. In fact, the components of the place may have some interesting aspects that relate to the individual's symbology, which are projections of his or her needs. For example, some "places" are filled with nature's elements, like trees and rocks, while others may contain human elements, like beds and chairs.

4. **Determining the median of wisdom:** Although the elements of nature (ocean, sun, moon, etc.) may deliver messages to the individual, usually there is a person or animal that can communicate information to the person on the visual quest. Sometimes this entity is a recognized person, like a grandparent or a spiritual figure, but more often than not it is a being with a combination of traits that convey wisdom and clarity for the person. These traits may be represented in a strange contortion of characteristics, like an entity with a face of a person, a body of a dog and wings of a bird. The basic understanding is that this figure is not part of ordinary reality, so the appearance does not have to conform to ordinary life as we know it. The entity may communicate to the person directly or by other means, or may not communicate at all. This may mean that the person's mission or question is not appropriate at this time or needs to be re-examined for more specificity.

Once the question has been addressed in some fashion, the entity will leave, even if the individual is not satisfied.

5. **Returning:** Generally returning to ordinary reality is the easiest part. It is recommended that the person return the same way he or she departed, such as through the sky or through the earth, in order to complete a trip. There is a sense of safety in returning over the way one comes.

6. **Re-considering the question or the mission:** Sometimes the answers take a long time to understand; the meanings may be so symbolic that the communications are confusing. For example, one person asked whether or not his power as a person would continue after a surgical operation. His particular entity began laughing and continued laughing throughout the experience. The person was puzzled, but after a month of contemplation he reasoned that the answer was laughable. After all, the part of his body to be modified, in fact his whole body, had nothing to do with his power as a person, his essence of self. He laughed at his question himself.

The vision quest imagery journey is not a new approach to finding the answers to life's questions. All spiritual leaders have gone on vision quests to help formulate their respective missions in the world. However, the answers are not easy to understand and may not ever be fully understood. Sometimes it is the process that is most helpful—the process of the struggle and the experience of being in the presence of "the place" that is most comforting.

The Mythic Hero's Journey

In the mythic hero's journey, there is always the possibility of error, since we have not been given a map of life. Perhaps that is the role of the storyteller, to give hope and some assistance in the next step. In any uncertain journey, we will be led into directions in which we make errors; hopefully we learn from one step to the next. All too often, critics emerge who undermine our confidence, especially as we are struggling with the greatest questions of our lives.

The Cure is about cure and transformation but not about total restoration to the state of health before disease. Alex is not the same as before; we are left with the possibility that he may actually be better than he was before the disease. At least he has come to a better understanding of the essence of what his life is. The task of the journey is not to return to where we began but go further into our own self-understanding.

There will be errors on the journey, but there will be no mistakes. Errors are simply processes by which we learn that we can make other choices that will likely have better outcomes. Errors are always learning opportunities. Mistakes are those choices that we should not have made or that we regret. Since we learn more from our errors than from our successes, we should never begrudge a person for making an error or deny a person the opportunity for making an error, for he or she should hopefully learn something from it. But whether the person makes a mistake—who is to tell, unless nothing can be learned from it.

This story has nothing to do with giving "false hope." Offering hope is supporting a person to explore possibilities. Occasionally someone will accuse me of giving people the false impression that they may live longer than expected if they use imagery and relaxation. Actually, my belief is that length of life becomes irrelevant to the quality of life and the wonderful challenge that confronts all of us—the ultimate understanding of who we are, and the discovery of what we can be.

Alex made a few of these discoveries about himself, but his story is not necessarily anyone else's. What Alex has done is blaze a path so that we can better understand the courage needed to continue on our personal vision quest and to search for the basic compass within ourselves.

4. Self-Empowerment: The Warrior-Self

Regardless of the techniques used, the primary goal of *The Cure* is to help listeners discover self-empowerment, an attribute difficult to obtain while experiencing the medical care system. We have discussed three ways of how caregivers may help listeners empower themselves.

- Relaxation and imagery can help listeners gain management over pain, nausea and anxiety.

- Using power symbols can help listeners focus on participating in disease management.

- Educating listeners about the disease gives perspective on intervention strategies.

Self-empowerment usually evolves from these efforts to develop a participatory relationship between the patient and the disease. One setback to self-empowerment is that the term "patient" almost inherently implies the "victim" concept. As an adjective, "patient" is defined as "enduring pain, trouble, etc., without complaint"[1]; as a noun, the word's meaning connotes receiving medical treatment in a passive manner. In the last century, the discovery of invisible (to the naked eye) agents—germs, virus and bacteria—has created a cloak of secrecy or a sense of mystery about the nature of disease. Perhaps not unlike the previous theories of invisible demons and disease, only those with the correct "vision" (in present cases, those with microscopes, X-rays, MRIs, etc.) are capable of discovering these agents and therefore are the only ones able to correct the problems. These marvelous devices have helped develop our understanding of health, no doubt, but one of the results of such procedures is the isolation the person with the disease feels. No longer are his or her feelings discussed in light of the diagnosis. The person becomes a set of organs—a couple of lungs, a heart, etc.

However, the definition of "medicine" is "to make whole," to return to harmony and balance. However sophisticated the technology, the spirit of the person whose life has been disrupted also needs to be made whole again. In order to accomplish this task, which is unique to each individual, the person must become a participant in the healing journey. The major cause of disease or complications from disease is loneliness, regardless of the diagnosis, because of isolation from sources of energetic support outside the medical realm. It is difficult to assert one's needs, especially emotional

---

[1] *American Heritage Dictionary* (New York: Dell, 1983).

ones, in a world of intense focus upon the physical process of disease, with little or no focus upon the accompanying mental suffering.

Again, this is not an indictment of the medical profession; it is a concern for the person to overcome these obstacles. Perhaps the person can benefit from giving consideration to the obstacles of the health system; such consideration may help the person find the courage and resources to rise to the occasion of being a warrior for self—keeping in mind, however, that the healthcare system is not the focus of attack.

The concept of the warrior-self emerges from the mythic stories of the warrior-hero, in which a person is challenged for honor's sake. From the new research on multiple consciousness, we have found that within each of us is a warrior consciousness that emerges under the right circumstances. The normally passive mother becomes outraged and aggressive when her children are threatened. The normally quiet man turns into a soldier when he hears that his nation is being fired upon. Each of us has the capability of becoming a warrior, but, probably because of the our culture's values and lack of appropriate need to do so, we tend to suppress it most of our lives.

The Cure focuses upon one issue of life and the process of realizing our need for self-nurturing and protection. However, many other life issues besides disease require that we undergo similar transformative processes in order to understand and cope with them. Following are some of the major issues that usually accompany our life struggle:

- Life changes and skill demands
- Belief changes

- Life-stage changes
- Life-rhythm changes
- Work changes
- Relationship changes
- Physical stamina changes

Life Changes and Skill Demands

Life changes are those changes that occur at any time in our living experience and that cause us to develop a new skill of adaptation and coping. For example, there is the change of moving to a new home or having new neighbors. There may be few things to change, but new things to learn—perhaps new languages, new customs and even new surroundings. Stories of new beginnings are often helpful during these times, especially if they relate to actual specific situations.

Belief Changes

Belief changes are those made when a basic belief is severely challenged. One challenge to our beliefs that we often meet with great resistance is a change in our perception of parents—that they are human and not God-like or perfect. This realization becomes only too real during adolescence. We also face changes in perception about ourselves as we have significant experiences in this regard. Stories about the basic validity of values and stable perceptions have special meaningfulness during these times, even for adults.

Life-Stage Changes

Life stages are those eventual processes, both physical and social, which occur in all people's lives: childhood, adulthood, parenthood, middle age, older age. These phases are part of growing older and gaining experience. Except for a few transitional phases, like birth, marriage and maybe reaching adulthood, very few of these transformations are honored with ritual and meaningfulness. It is recommended that the process of these life-stage developments be met with some support and stories that communicate an appropriate path in these times of change.

Life-Rhythm Changes

Life rhythms are the times of change in our usual routine, such as those that result from the new responsibilities of having a child or getting a pet. Obviously, some of these changes may not be eventful, but many are. Finding the meaningfulness of the experience can make the process a positive and a healthy one. Vision quest stories are often helpful in this regard.

Work Changes

Work change is recognized as the change of responsibilities, expectations and roles that accompany vocational life. Of course, a major work change is retirement; but during our work life we experience a multitude of changes that come every two or three years, such as transitions of supervisors, of supervisees, of markets, etc.

Work can serve as a valuable aspect of stability in our lives, especially since most people's welfare depends upon the generated income. However, many people develop self-esteem from their work. For example, some will introduce themselves as what they do as a worker— "I am a secretary," or lawyer, executive, etc.—or as part of the production process—"I am an assistant to the president of Acme Milling Company, making 100,000 mills a day." If disease becomes prohibitive to these people's identity as workers, they may begin to question their personal worth.

Relationship Changes

Probably no major threat to the sense of essence or self is as great as the impact of interpersonal relationships, whether it be family, lover, close friends or community at large. The costs of isolation and exile often experienced in these relationships are great in terms of emotional as well as physical accounts. Included within the realm of interpersonal change is the process of grief over loss through death, geographical distance or personal separation decisions such as divorce. The process of grief must be honored as a way of giving credence to the existence of the relationship, the integrity of its development and how important it served the persons involved.

Death or loss is a natural phenomenon that will probably occur in everyone's lifetime; it is a time for reflection on the relationship with that person as well as on the added quality of life as a result of having a relationship. However, to cut short the process of healing that a grief period allows is to cut short the process of giving honor to that relationship. In this process, it is very important to engage symbols and memorials within a story to aid in this understanding and conclusion.

Physical Stamina Changes

"Physical stamina" is a general term for loss of youth, or what our culture refers to as sexuality and beauty. As in the discussion about overidentifying with our work, many of us have the notion that we are our bodies. Yet the majority of the citizens of the United States believe in the existence of a more permanent part of our character—the soul. We need to be reminded of that essence of ourselves that is not embedded in the physical decay of the body. The journey part of the imaged vision quest helps us understand that separation between body and soul and the multi-faceted definition of who we are. We can be anything and bring forth whatever persona we wish to present to the world.

Being a warrior for self does not mean being an attacker of another person or institution. It is an attitude, a state of mind that is a centered and grounded sense of self in the present tense. In essence, the warrior-self's attitude is that character and intent in whatever happens are the primary, if not the only, values. No future or past events should take energy. The past is gone, and no one can predict the future anyway, so the present is all we know.

The warrior philosophy comes from the fact that, as a warrior, all wars should be honorable and the next battle may be the last. The worst possibility is to die with regret or cowardice; therefore, at any moment one must be prepared to live as if that moment were the last. Since death is an ultimate reality for all of us, the warrior is concerned with *how* he or she lives life, not for *how long*.

As warriors, the challenge is to be our authentic self, the self truest to our convictions as if there were no future. The warrior-self role takes courage and tremendous strength to maintain our authentic self in the face of the forces that diminish our self-empowerment.

In the story, Alex realizes that his warrior-self has not been present and that he has given away his power in his fear and confusion. He resolves to return to the doctor animals of the forest with his warrior-self concept and maintain a participatory relationship. In his process of allowing the power of self to emerge, his healing begins.

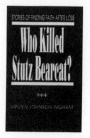

WHO KILLED STUTZ BEARCAT?
Stories of Finding Faith after Loss

Kristen Johnson Ingram

Paper, $8.95, 0-89390-264-0

Nine stories encourage readers to find courage within themselves after facing losses. Reflection questions will lead readers beyond the author's stories and into their own. As readers reflect upon personal experiences, they may discover their own possibilities for resurrection. This book is appropriate for grief ministry work, pastoral counseling, initiation groups, or individual reflection.

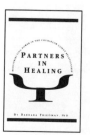

PARTNERS IN HEALING
Redistributing Power in the Counselor-Client Relationship

Barbara Friedman, PhD

Paper, $14.95, 0-89390-226-8

The traditional therapy model requires one person to have power over another. That's trouble, says Dr. Barbara Friedman, herself a practicing psychologist. With this book, she proposes a therapeutic model in which counselor and client interact as equal partners in the healing process. This unique book is must reading for therapists, clergy and pastoral counselors, lay counselors, and clients.

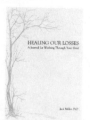

HEALING OUR LOSSES
A Journal for Working Through Your Grief

Jack Miller, PhD

Paper, $10.95, 0-89390-255-1

The author shares experiences of loss in his own life and guides you to record memories, thoughts, and feelings about loss in your life. This book offers comfort to anyone grieving a loss and can help eventually heal the pain. The process may be used by an individual or in a group setting.

Improve Your Storytelling Skills!

STORYTELLING STEP-BY-STEP

Marsh Cassady, PhD

Paper, $9.95
0-89390-183-0

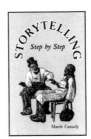

Marsh Cassady, a storytelling and drama instructor, takes you through all the steps of storytelling: selecting the right story for your audience, adapting your story for different occasions, analyzing it to determine the best way to present it, preparing your audience, and presenting the story. Includes many story examples.

CREATING STORIES FOR STORYTELLING

Marsh Cassady, PhD

Paper, $9.95
0-89390-205-5

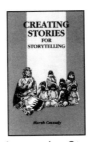

This book picks up where the author's popular *Storytelling Step-by-Step* leaves off. Find out how to get ideas to create your own original stories, adapt stories to different audiences, plot a story, create tension, and write dialogue.

Order Form

Order these resources from your local bookstore, or mail this form to:

QTY	TITLE	PRICE	TOTAL

Subtotal: _____

CA residents add 7¼% sales tax
(Santa Clara Co. residents, 8¼%): _____

Postage and handling
($2 for order to $20; 10% of order over $20 but
less than $150; $15 for order of $150 or more): _____

Total: _____

Resource Publications, Inc.
160 E. Virginia Street #290 - B7
San Jose, CA 95112-5876
(408) 286-8505
(408) 287-8748 FAX

☐ My check or money order is enclosed.

☐ Charge my ☐ VISA ☐ MC.

Expiration Date _____

Card # _____ - _____ -_____ - _____

Signature _____

Name (print)_____

Institution _____

Street_____

City/State/ZIP _____